The Mother's Guide to the Meaning of Life

What Being a Mom Has Taught Me about Resiliency, Guilt, Acceptance, and Love

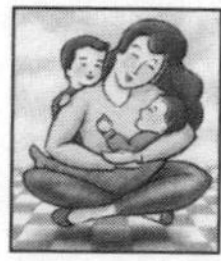

By Amy Krouse Rosenthal

author of *The Book of Eleven*
and creator of *www.mommymommy.com*

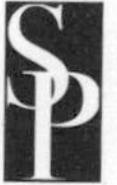

Skyhorse Publishing

Published by arrangement with Rodale, Inc.

Skyhorse Publishing books may be purchased in bulk at special discounts for sales promotion, corporate gifts, fund-raising, or educational purposes. Special editions can also be created to specifications. For details, contact the Special Sales Department, Skyhorse Publishing, 307 West 36th Street, 11th Floor, New York, NY 10018 or info@skyhorsepublishing.com.

www.skyhorsepublishing.com

10 9 8 7 6 5 4 3 2

Library of Congress Cataloging-in-Publication Data is available on file.
ISBN: 978-1-51073-103-5

Printed in China

The MOTHER'S GUIDE to the MEANING of LIFE

Titles in the

Guides to the Meaning of Life

series

The Father's Guide to the Meaning of Life

The Mother's Guide to the Meaning of Life

The Runner's Guide to the Meaning of Life

The Golfer's Guide to the Meaning of Life

For Jason, my partner,
my Saint (of Maxime)

Contents

Acknowledgments

I'd like to thank manuscript readers Ann Wolk Krouse, Paul Krouse, Beth Kaufmann, Katie Froelich, Cindy Kaplan, Lindy Hirschsohn, and Jason Rosenthal; Rodaleians Susan Clarey, Neil Wertheimer, Lisa Andruscavage, and Renee James; children Justin, Miles, and Paris; contributors Renee Raab Whitcombe, Wendy Abrams, Daniel Spatucci, Barb Cooke, Virginia Halstead; assistants Celine Chary and Laura Dzbinski; spirit lifters Howard Gossage, Sophie Calle, James Thurber, Kathy Hepinstall, Andy Kaufman, Masahide ("The barn's burnt down, now I can see the moon"), Michael Glab, and Katerina's Coffeehouse in Chicago; lovely children Justin, Miles, and Paris; WBEZ people Justin Kaufmann and Cate Cahan; Thursday girl Charise Mericle Harper; agent Amy Rennert; mommy-mommy.com queen Marya Smith; "propellers" Chip Rowe, Cathie Walker, Dave Eggers, Neil Genzlinger, Marcia Menter, Dave Slipp, Michael Rosen, Anne Dalin, Mark Bazer, Patrick Regan, and Stephanie Bennett; meaning-of-life suppliers Justin, Miles, and Paris.

Cast of Characters

Justin .... age 7, likes his oranges peeled and sectioned

Miles .... age 5, likes his oranges quartered, skin on

Paris .... age 3, likes her oranges cut vertically, in circles

Jason .... also known as Dad; calm, wise, and easygoing; likes his oranges any old way

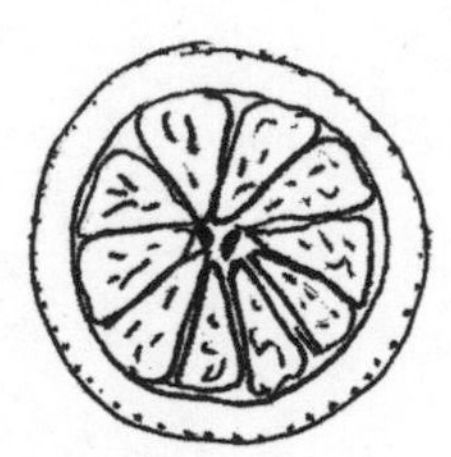

introduction

Go

PUTTING AN END TO NOT STARTING

Before our first child, Justin, was born, I had never changed a diaper in my life. I was really nervous about this. How can I possibly have a baby if I have no clue how those little diaper tabs work? Like millions of women before me, I walked into the hospital bloated and diaper-challenged and walked out still a bit bloated but a diaper guru. Just like that. Two or three changings and I had it covered, so to speak.

We parents figure it out because we have to. Not figuring it out is not an option.

Whether one is starting a family, starting a book, or starting a revolution, there is never a shortage of reasons not to start. *I can't start until I have it all figured out, until we buy a house, until my shipment of megaphones comes in.* There's always some glitch, some delay, something that we convince ourselves needs to happen before we can officially begin.

Only two problems with this logic:

1. The down-the-road route may very well prove to have even more potholes than it does now.
2. Who's to say there will even *be* a down the road? Who's to say I won't walk out the door at 4:29 this afternoon, take two steps to my left, wave "hi" to my neighbor Marya, and then get flattened by a falling air conditioner?

Just as there never seems to be a good time to start something major, there never seems to be a shortage of people who believe that they are authorities on good and bad timing. I had the pleasure of meeting some of these insightful people when I graduated from college and was trying to get a job.

They kept telling me, "Now is the worst possible time to find a job. The market is just awful." What does that *mean*? What does that have to do with *anything*? It's always a bad time. People always say that. That is the most un-useful information I ever heard, and it certainly didn't have anything at all to do with my reality.

The only reality for me was that I had to get a job and that I would have to interview daily, in uncomfortable shoes, until I found one. If I had waited until it was a "good" time, I'd still be hanging out in my folks' family room, greeting them when they came home from work with a Cheetos-stained piece of paper. "Hey, look guys—great news: I got another letter today from my pen pal Ted Kaczynski!"

***

The best time to plant a tree is 20 years ago.
The second best time is today.

—Proverb

(The best time to change a stinky diaper is 20 minutes ago.
The second best time is this minute.)

Today, I still do not have it all figured out. I possess neither tantrum-free children nor a Ph.D.* For these reasons and so many more, it makes absolutely perfect sense for me to *not* start this book. I should wait until the book is all mapped out in my head; I should wait until the new, updated thesaurus comes out; I should wait until I've read every classic, or at least one of them; I should wait until I learn every single thing there is to learn and think every single thought there is to think.

Indeed it would behoove all involved if, prior to starting, I would spend some time evolving over the course of five or six more lifetimes, until I came back finally as the world's first fully evolved, highly enlightened Dalai Mama. But I'm not sure if my contract has a provision for that sort of thing. ■

*Please note that the only Ph.D. I have is the one all parents have, and it stands for Putting in Hours Daily.

P.S. I know your mind is going to wander, that despite my best efforts and countless hours looking for the perfect metaphor ("like a Zamboni"), you will find yourself rereading the same paragraph four times because the only thing on your mind is "Green Giant teriyaki vegetables, don't forget Green Giant teriyaki vegetables for dinner." And because nearly every book I own is missing the first, mostly-blank title page due to some errand-on-the-brain casualty, you'll note the blank pages in the back of the book for your grocery list, punchlist for the contractor, questions for your child's upcoming parent/teacher conference. Use them, tear them out, clear your mind of all the lint that's preventing you from hanging on to my every word.

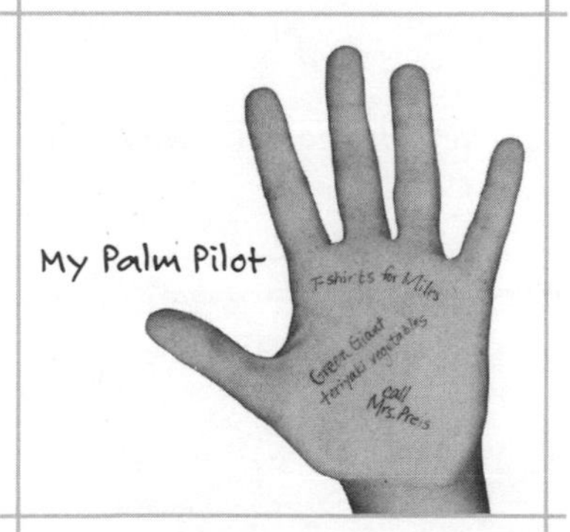
My Palm Pilot
T-shirts for Miles
Green Giant teriyaki vegetables
Call Mrs. Preis

insight

Words That Move a Mother

1. *My house is clean enough to be healthy, and messy enough to be happy.*

—ANONYMOUS

2. *I tried to allow my children to take risks,*
to test themselves. Better broken bones, than
broken spirit.

—ROSE KENNEDY

3. *She asked me if I had kids and when I said I did she said, make sure you teach them what's right and I said, how will I know? And she nodded and said, good point, just don't teach them any obvious wrong then.*

—BRIAN ANDREAS
artist

4. If We'd Wanted Quiet, We Would Have Raised Goldfish.

—BRUCE LANSKY
title of anthology
of poems for parents

5. *Little girls, and little boys*
your world is filled with many joys:
music, laughter,
the sound of rain;
kinship, cupcakes,
a lion's mane;
Mozart, Beaux Arts, Humphrey Bogart,
fish in the bay . . .
_______________ *, (insert your child[ren]'s name)*
let us give thanks for this new day.

—ANONYMOUS

6. *It's frightening to think that you mark your children merely by being yourself. . . . It seems unfair. You can't assume the responsibility for everything you do—or don't do.*

—SIMONE DE BEAUVOIR

Les Belles Images

7. Your responsibility as a parent is not as great as you might imagine. You need not supply the world with the next conqueror of disease or major motion-picture star. If your child simply grows up to be someone who does not use the word "collectible" as a noun, you can consider yourself an unqualified success.

—FRAN LEBOWITZ
Social Studies

8. She discovered with great delight that one does not love one's children just because they are one's children but because of the friendship formed while raising them.

—GABRIEL GARCÍA MÁRQUEZ
Love in the Time of Cholera

9. Maybe my cup is too full.

—VIRGINIA HALSTEAD

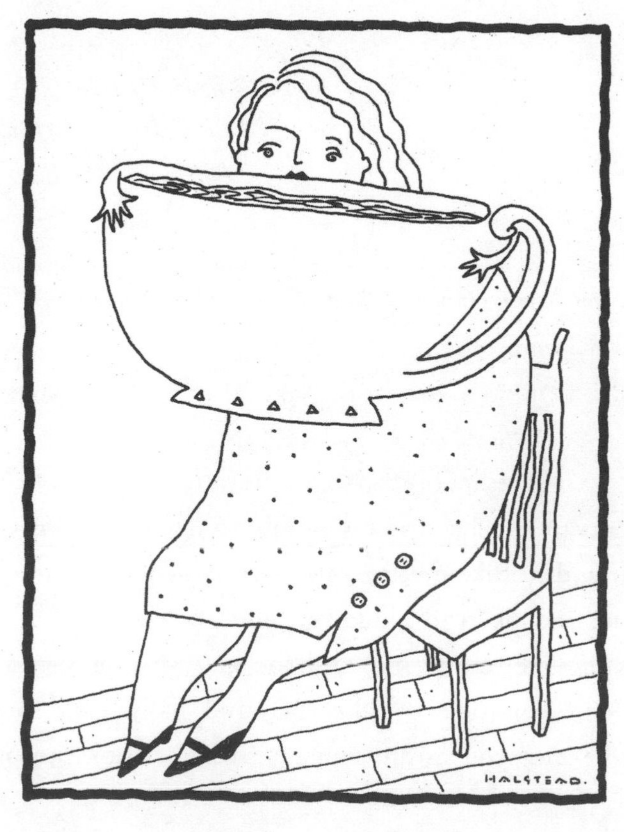

lesson one

Such a Nice Chapter

ON DISPLEASING SOME OF THE PEOPLE SOME OF THE TIME

If you have never been hated by your child, you have never been a parent.

—Bette Davis

For someone who wants not only my parents to like me, and my family to like me, and my friends to like me, but also people who don't like me to convert to liking me, and people who don't know me to like me, and the guy who delivered our Thai food to like me, and Sally Field to like me, you might imagine that it took me a while to be okay with the fact that my kids are not going to like me all the time.

> The first time I had to fill out a form for preschool, in the space for MOTHER: ________, I wrote Ann, my mom's name. I then realized that, wait, they mean me, I'm the mother now.

Not worrying about being nice, like understanding cilantro, is something I grew into. Though I've made great bitch headway, I still find myself with the need to end on a good note. For example, let's say we had a horrid drive to school—the kids were bickering, someone forgot his backpack, they're at their annoying zenith. When they're piling out of the car, I still feel compelled to insert a pause, then a perky, "Have a great day! I love you!"

I am certain that my kids really want me to be mean sometimes. They want to be assured that their parents are not wimps. They're just double-checking, yep, cool, mom has a spine. Not only that, but children have an amazing capacity to move on from being mad. That's the big secret. Small children forget that they're mad. You actually have to remind them! *Don't draw a picture of a heart and flowers for me—you are mad at me, remember?* They haven't mastered the art of pouting like we do. Their capacity to hold a grudge is in direct proportion to how high they can count: So that's what—11 seconds? 29? 214 for a gifted preschooler?

And worst-case scenario: What if, as they get older, as their memory skills increase, they are able to sustain their disdain? So they don't think we're nice for a few minutes—or days—here or there? Fantastic! Erma Bombeck used to say that if you're lucky enough to have your kid mad at you, take advantage of it and go on vacation. Use up those free miles.

Those times that I did put one of the kids to sleep upset, meaning I didn't wait for him to settle down and be pleased with me before we parted our nocturnal ways, I would be sure that he woke up seething with hatred for me; that, in fact, his hatred, having marinated overnight, would have intensified into a robust loathing mixed with disappointment, disgust, and pity, and he would no longer be a happy little child but rather that kind of adult-child who clearly has had his innocence prematurely, violently ripped away and has become, in that one instant, wise, quiet, and sad. This episode right here, with my leaving him screaming in his room, would be the precise moment that everything changed for us, no way for mother and child to go back and undo the psychological trauma of it all. This would be his plight, his load, and it would be rehashed many times over the years, with his understanding aunt, with his buddies in college, with his therapist on the ninth floor of a gray building downtown whose waiting room is full of back issues of *U.S. News and World Report.*

But then:

"Ma-a-a-a-a-a-u-u-u-u-u-umme-e-e-e-e-e-e-e-e!"
Is that a happy person calling me?

" Ma-a-a-a-a-a-u-u-u-u-umme-e-e-e-e-e-e-e-e."
I go to his crib. There he is, beaming as always, with outstretched arms.

You'd think, out of common courtesy, he could have at least faked a half-(diaper)assed grudge. ■

insight

The Essential Traits of a Mother

1. LAP—The three most important and completely obvious traits happen to form the fitting acronym LAP: Love, the Ability to get by on little or no sleep, and Patience.
2. Humility—First of all, how much of our child's being and persona can we rightfully claim is due to our fabulous influence: 20 percent, 14 percent, 1 percent? So much of who they are is just who they are, so taking credit or modestly flicking it away is irrelevant. Nonetheless, we're human, and we can't help thinking that all our hard work and sticker charts add up to something; that our efforts deserve to be publicly noted and commended—a full-blown parade would be nice. Even so, we parents must always be humble. Because to boast about your well-mannered angel is to seal the fate that within 40 seconds, he will be peeing on your neighbor's tulips.
3. Perspective—My friend Jeff says a good day is when everything's working: The car is working, the house is working, things at the kids' school are working, he's

working. No major glitches equals an awesome day. Ear infections, flat tires, baseball mitts left at playgrounds, cabinet doors falling off their hinges—they are nuisances, nothing more, nothing less.

4. Intuition—It's that vague yet undeniable inner twitch, that palpable gurgle of meaning we hear in the silence, detect in the offbeat, see in the blackness. It's how you know something's off with the babysitter (she's scratching her nose again; every time I ask her about the park, she scratches her nose). It's how you know that your child is sick before she's sick. It's how you wake up in the middle of the night 20 seconds before the hungry whimpers of your newborn set in. It's how you know something is wrong with the car even though it's technically driving "fine." It's how you know that this time your child needs a severe punishment, not just a time-out. It's how my mom knew in eighth grade that P. was not my cool new friend but a gal with a beau-stealing plan. Intuition travels up through the gut

and out of the mouth in the form of the words, "I don't know—I just *know*."

5. Sense of humor—a) You're driving across Florida with three small children and zero cold beverages and get caught in Phish concert traffic—to be exact, 2 hours of bumper-to-bumper 19-year-olds. *How funny! Ha, ha, ha.*

   b) You've just broken the last remaining champagne flute from your bridal registry when your toddler calls you over to see the entire roll of toilet paper that "fell" into the toilet, and your son says, "Oh, this is for you," and hands you a school flyer warning of a lice breakout. *Ha, ha, hysterical—more, please, more!*

   c) You walk out of the real estate closing and realize that you had a Tarzan sticker stuck to your left breast. *Funny stuff.*

   If you have a really good sense of humor, you can laugh at this kind of stuff as it's unfolding. The rest of us need the distance of a day or two to realize, oh yeah, that was actually pretty funny.

6. Multi-tasking—It's how you're able to hand out the goodie bags at the birthday party while wrapping up leftover cake for your husband's grandmother while finalizing tomorrow's car pool details with Jacob's mom. It explains why your grocery list has cryptic notes in the margin like:

   - M's sympathy note
   - meeting/soup analogy
   - teacher gifts – lavender?

   It's why you think it's normal that you are simultaneously slicing flank steak, helping your daughter decorate a sombrero for Crazy Hat Day, and reading this book.

7. The ability to ask for help—To wit, I asked my e-pal Laurie Feinswog what she thought were the essential traits of a mother. Here's her smart and lovely response. Mothers must have a) good diplomatic skills, e.g., able to see the child's side at school,

the teacher's side at home; b) unconditional love, in spite of the Sharpie marker left open on the new couch; c) the courage to ask a stranger to help you carry a bag of groceries; d) mathematic prowess, or at least be comfortable counting in fractional increments: "I'm warning you . . . One, two, two-and-a-half, TWO-AND-THREE-QUARTERS . . . ; and e) self-forgiveness.

8. Time management—I know this is an essential trait because I do not possess it, and I'm constantly paying the consequences. I'm baffled, daily, by my complete inability to properly gauge what can and cannot be accomplished inside an hour. I think I can miraculously alter time, that the system is flexible, that, for example, if I get on the treadmill at 5:37 and want to get in a 30-minute run but have to be done by 6 o'clock, I can actually outrun the 30 minutes. The laws of space and time aren't really set in stone. I have an inkling that, if I hurry, if I concentrate, I can make 30 minutes out of 20.

Exhibit A: ***A Simple Thing Never Takes Just 2 Minutes***

7 minutes talking about doing that thing
4 minutes reminding the kids that we are going to do that thing
4 minutes looking for lost items (misplaced cheetah toy that child must have this instant; barrette daughter just dropped in between couch cushions) postpones doing that thing
3 minutes taking a phone call from sister further delays doing that thing
2 minutes actually doing that thing
20 minutes total

9. Resiliency—To be a mom is to have, at any given moment, everything turned completely on its head. That is why the word for Mom is Mom and not Som or Pom or Bloot—because MOM upside down is WOW. That is it right there, the single truth, inherent in the very word—motherhood is one, big, intense, erratic, emphatic WOW. Wow, this is tough! Wow, this is joyous! Wow, this is a nightmare! Wow, this is phenomenal! Wow, I love these kids! Wow, are they annoying!

World's Greatest
WoW

lesson two

Running Away

ARE YOU STILL A GOOD MOTHER IF YOU FANTASIZE ABOUT BAILING FOR A FEW HOURS . . . OR YEARS?

The fantasy first presented itself during a conversation with my artist/truck driver friend Walter. "I'm hitting the road again," he told me one afternoon. This is his life—6 months escorting cargo cross-country, 6 months back at home making art.

Here's what went through my mind in about 1.8 seconds: I could see Walter sitting in the driver's seat, his paint-stained hands on the enormous wheel; pan right over to the passenger seat, and there's . . . me! Backpack tucked at my ankles, pen in hand, journal on lap. I am tagging along, mile after dusty

I have little patience for figuring out how a package or bag of lettuce opens. I typically tear right into it instead of taking a moment to assess the opening options, and realize only after the fact, that, yes, right here is a nice perforated line or TEAR HERE arrow that would have made opening it much easier and much neater.

mile, writing all sorts of great, masterful things and eating all sorts of bad, salty things. It is a glorious, pivotal time of my life. Can you hear us jamming to Lenny Kravitz? . . . *I want to run away, I want to flyyyyyyyy away. . . .*

Then, around the 1.9th second, the fantasy was interrupted. "Excuse me, over here, on your other shoulder. Quick reminder: You have a husband, three small children, and one very large to-do list; you're not going anywhere. Now, weren't you about to throw a Bounce sheet into the dryer?"

What intrigued me was the fact that I had had this fantasy at all. I mean, I love my kids. I love my husband, except when he forgets to give me phone messages. I love our broken little house. And if the right music is playing and the rain is falling just so and I'm feeling too melancholy for my own good, even the most mundane domestic detail can seem pleasing—like, say, the fridge cluttered with the kids' artwork, snapshots, and an assortment of cheesy, promotional magnets. In short, I like my life way more than I like road trips.

So why the fantasy? Am I despicable for having had it? To find out, I did what any respectable American reared on guilt and talk shows would do: I tracked down a couple of celebrity therapists.

***

A Beverly Hills clinical psychologist by the name of Dr. Judy was the first to bring the good news: I tested normal! She told me that until we have kids, we are more or less in a self-serving state. Then Baby arrives and breaks up the big me-fest. She says that the fantasy of running away is useful and healthy because it helps prevent the mother from acting out her impulses. Case in point: The subject is writing this from her home office, not from an 18-wheeler.

As you might recall, the expression "Misery loves company" was coined in 1748 by a sleep-deprived mother. In other words, I was thrilled to hear just how common the fantasy is. Harriet Lerner, Ph.D., author of *The Mother Dance: How Children Change Your Life*, says of course mothers want to flee when we consider the unrealistic expectations, the enormous amount of responsibility, and the sacrifice that is rarely equally shared by another adult. Thank you. Indeed, raising kids is a mother of a job. And it's tough even when you have major forces—such as a mate, financial stability, relatives in town—working in your favor. For those moms who have little or none of the above support, the flee fantasy is even more understandable. Clearly, it *does* take a village. And a lot of coffee.

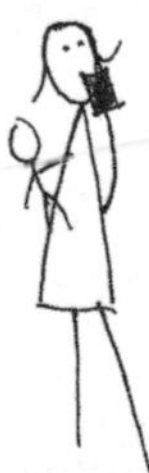

Mother with child and latté

So what are we to do? Dr. Lerner prescribes the following:

1. Understand that these feelings are totally normal. We need to lose the guilt; most of us are struggling from one hour to the next. And you know those moms who have "easy" children? Don't speak to them.
2. Connect with other mothers. Do this early on, like, say, the minute the epidural wears off.
3. Gather all the support you can. "Self-sufficiency is the archenemy of mothers everywhere," warns Dr. Lerner. As with doing the *New York Times* crossword puzzle, no one expects you to do it single-handedly. Seek and accept the help of others.
4. Let go of perfectionism. Just drop it. And look at it this way: If you really were a perfect mother, everyone would hate you.

I always imagined that all the other, better mothers were swiftly gliding through parenthood and would never, oh my never!, feel like bolting. Our culture does a pretty good job of presenting motherhood as this blissful, downy-soft state of being, and so we feel guilty and ashamed when what we actually feel inside—bliss, yes, but also frustration, exhaustion, occasional nausea—doesn't exactly match the manufactured illusion. "For how beautiful and powerful and wonderful motherhood is, there is pain," Anne Stoline, a Baltimore psychiatrist specializing in women's mental health, told me. "It requires constant growth and vigilance. And women who are able to maintain their perspectives—perhaps partly through fantasizing—know that, ultimately, there is relief." Yes, now I see it . . . the light at the end of the McDonald's Playplace tunnel.

It's relentless, motherhood is. That's the most accurate way I can put it: relentless. Relentless in its demands, relentless in its joys. There is always one more car pool, one more tantrum over the wrong color sippy cup, one more birthday party to get a bright-plastic present for. Yet, God willing, there is always one more lopsided Popsicle-stick jewelry box, one more smile from across the park, one more chorus of "Mommy's home!" ■

insight

A Mother's Essential Reading

1. *GIFT FROM THE SEA* by Anne Morrow Lindbergh

From the perspective of a week away at the beach, a mother sorts out her full life and makes peace with its demands.

2. *EVERYONE'S A COACH* by Don Shula

Some fabulous coaching tactics that apply directly to parenting, from one of the all-time greats.

3. *PURE DRIVEL* by Steve Martin

When you need to laugh your head off.

4. *FOREVER, ERMA* by Erma Bombeck

Because no one said it better.

5. *PROTECTING THE GIFT* by Gavin De Becker

6. *RAISING AN EMOTIONALLY INTELLIGENT CHILD* by John Gottman, Ph.D.

7. THE AMERICAN MEDICAL ASSOCIATION FAMILY MEDICAL GUIDE

The big blue savior that's as much for the mental health of a mother as it is for the physical health of her child.

Diagnosis According to a Mother's Mind

Child has a runny nose	brain tumor
Child has a headache	brain tumor
Child has a funny spot on arm . . .	arm tumor
Everything else	rare, fatal disease

Diagnosis According to the AMA

Child has a runny nose	nasal discharge can be a sign of a cold
Child has a headache	headache is a common symptom of a cold
Child has a funny spot on arm . . .	a hair follicle may have become infected

8. "IN PRAISE OF BOREDOM" Originally a commencement address at Dartmouth from *On Grief and Reason* by Joseph Brodsky, winner of the Nobel Prize for literature in 1987.

9. Mostly, to stay sane, read anything that's precisely not about motherhood. Some favorites include:

THE PILLOW BOOK by Sei Shonagon

TIME OUT OF MIND by Leonard Michaels

HOW PROUST CAN CHANGE YOUR LIFE by Alain De Botton

CDB! by William Steig

LOST IN THE FUNHOUSE by Bill Zehme

THE NEW NEW THING by Michael Lewis

A HEARTBREAKING WORK OF STAGGERING GENIUS by Dave Eggers

BIRDS OF AMERICA by Lorrie Moore

Anything by Paul Auster

lesson three

Learning to Walk

AFTER 35 YEARS,
I'M LEARNING HOW

The Mister and I were away at a spa in Tuscon called Miravel, a place whose logo includes the words "Life in balance," which got me right there. The buzz at the spa was that something called Equine Experience was the class to take. Now I am not a horse person—I fell asleep during *The Horse Whisperer*, but everyone promised while, yes, you basically groomed horses, that it was much more—that you learn about yourself in a way you can't imagine. So, with great unenthusiasm, I signed up . . . then promptly blew it off the next morning when the time came. I almost escaped equineless, but on the eve of our departure, I collapsed under the pressure of the 87th person ranting about it. So I signed up for the 9:00 A.M. class on our last day, knowing that that would leave me about 4½ spare minutes before our noon pickup time. Which was good, cause I had had enough of this leisurely pace crap.

"I'm Wyatt," said a graying Marlboro-ish man. A couple of sentences later, it was clear that he was more of a Plato-ish man, with a dash of the Tootsie Pop wise old owl. I subsequently learned that Wyatt had dropped out of life for a good 5 years and basically read every book ever written. He had a few things to share.

Wyatt took the three of us, all women, to the ring. There was a large horse standing alongside the fence. Wyatt went into the center. "Now I am going to get the horse to start walking." And with that, the horse started walking.

Keep in mind that words mean nothing to a horse; Wyatt was communicating solely through body language. He explained that the horse picks up on and basically mirrors back our energy, our intentions.

"Now the horse will trot." And the horse began to trot.

"Now he will run." And the horse ran.

Then Wyatt brought the horse back down to a trot, then a walk, then a stop. We three spectators were awestruck, giddy. It was really a beautiful and powerful thing to have witnessed.

"Your turn," he said.

Body language? Here's what my body language was saying: "Please, God, let me go last." So first one, then the other, woman took center ring and, with Wyatt's gentle guidance, figured out how to shift her energy and turn her body ever so slightly to take the horse from stop to run and back. Each had difficulty with one aspect or another—one couldn't get the horse to budge at first—but with Wyatt's coaching, everyone more or less mastered the exercise.

Wyatt's gaze fell my way. I said a silent prayer:

Please let me be able to do this; please let the horse not run me over—I still want to see the new Woody Allen movie.

If kids get prizes in their cereal boxes, shouldn't moms get something, too?

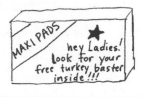

Wyatt showed me how to stand at a certain angle to the horse and how to adjust my wrist so the whip would dangle just so. And just like that, the horse started walking. Wow, no problem. Then he instructed me to think "trot" and turn ever so slightly. The horse started trotting. Cool. I'm really doing it. But then before Wyatt could okay the next level, and without my realizing what I had done, the horse was running. Running and running and running.

"Think trot," said Wyatt. And I tried to shift my energy back down and convey "trot" to this frantic creature. The horse responded. He began running even faster, like someone had laced his oats with a case of Dexatrim.

"All right, think walk, Amy. Walk. Walk. Walk,"

Wyatt said. I tried to think walk; to think slow; to be one with my loose, floppy shoulders; to think of taking a Sunday afternoon stroll while holding a bunny. But apparently my body language has a strong Chicago accent, because this horse was not understanding me one bit; he thought I was saying, "Run, freaky horse, run." After another minute or so—or maybe it was 6 days—of Wyatt's patient and pointed coaching, the horse finally, finally, finally settled into a trot, then a walk, then stopped.

Man.

I can say that at the time, this felt like one of the most profound lessons of my life, an image sure to make it into the final life-flashing-before-me slide show. I walked away with a clear agenda, a vow to mellow the hell out. Granted, within 20 minutes of being home, I blew all of that off. But I am able to catch myself now and again. I keep seeing the horse: running and running and running, and begging me to give him a break. ■

What If We Could Age Nonsequentially?

A CAMEO BY WENDY ABRAMS

Sometimes I wish we did not have to live our days sequentially. I mean, we all get the same number of days to live; you can't spend every day as a 20-year-old on spring break. But we shouldn't have to live them in order.

To be more specific, I am a 35-year-old mother of four. I spend my days changing diapers, washing bottles, brushing teeth, and (on a good day) brushing hair before rushing off to preschool or ballet or karate or all of the above. Cramped for time and short on energy, we stop at McDonald's, and I thank the person who invented drive-thru for saving me from having to unbuckle carseats and lug everyone inside. I'm the only one who really wants to take a nap. We paint, we swing, we play ball. Then it's back to carpooling, soccer practice, dinner, bath, and bed—a-a-ahh.

Ironically, it is not the days gone by that I had in mind when I stated this wish. For being 21 again does not provide me with anything that I do not already have (except maybe breasts). It is being 93, interspersed with 35, that I think would be tremendously valuable. For if I were 93, I admit, I would spend the first few hours of my day relishing the peace and quiet surrounding me. However, it would not be long before I would find myself sitting in the silence of my world, yearning to hear a child's voice, to hold a child's hand.

At 93, I would give all the treasures I had acquired through my many years of financial success, just to cuddle with that baby who simply wants me, just me. I would drag my tired bones up from my chair if that child asked to play with me. I would gladly walk to the park or just sit in the yard and watch for butterflies. There would be no place I had to go; no phone call worth interrupting this beautiful day. My slow pace and undivided attention would be all that this child required.

And then I would be 35 again, and I would be reminded that, in the end, what I will treasure most are my memories with my children. And I will feel as though those few chaotic years I spent in my thirties vanished in an instant. Returning from my day at 93, I know I will not regret spending less time out working or working out. I will reprioritize my life so that I will embrace the joys that are in front of me and I will be thankful for the good health with which I can enjoy them.

lesson four

(Mom)E-mail

A FRIEND IN NEED
IS A FRIEND ONLINE

The following e-mail correspondence with my pal Renee took place while she was in the midst of packing up her family and packing in her producer job in Los Angeles and moving to Cleveland for a couple of years for her husband's job.

From: amy krouse rosenthal <amy@suba.com>
Sent: april 3, 2000
To: "Renee Raab Whitcombe"
Subject: g

hi renee

Just finalized Paris's preschool plans for the fall. I'm sure we made the right decision—or, rather, every 4th day I'm sure. The other 3 days I'm sure of nothing.

Forget big decisions like school; even the small and inconsequential have the power to snag me. Like: I didn't sign Justin up for soccer, maybe I should have, even though he's expressed zero interest in it. Or I go to someone's house and see their toy room and realize we're the "bad toy house," that the few toys we do have totally suck, that I am depriving my children of fun board games, markers that aren't dried out, and bio-friendly wooden horses.

Maybe I need to bag city life and move to a farm... But then, I might have a hard time deciding what to grow—Corn? Strawberries? Artichokes?
> love,
> amy

From: "Renee Raab Whitcombe"
Sent: Mon, 10 Apr 2000 20:56:44 -0700
To: amy krouse rosenthal <amy@suba.com>
Subject: Re: g

Dear Amy,

I know a farm about 14 miles outside Cleveland . . .

It's funny to hear you say that, because here I go to the farm, and I'm not sure I'm thinking it's the ideal thing right now. It rocks my personal identity, to go from LA producer/woman/mom/person with friends and a place in my community, to new gal in the deep Midwest, aka Mike's wife and Alex's mom, you know, the pregnant woman from California.

I DO relate to what you were saying in that I am frantically running around our immediate area touring and applying to nursery schools for winter 2002, so Alex has a place to go when she is more than twice her current age. What if I am just rushing and get on the wrong waiting lists (which I am supposed to feel so lucky to be on)? What if a new, awesome preschool opens up after we leave, and I don't even KNOW about it till it's too late? And then I remind myself that I don't personally remember anything before I was 5 or 6.

I think we have to trust that we really are doing right by our kids, even though we're not always going to score the best piece of birthday cake, the corner piece with a candle *and* a flower. Because you make decisions based on the facts at the time, and you can't always know everything before you have to jump in and say, "I pick this." Besides, doesn't it just seem like we probably will get most of what is needed in the respectable realm of right?

I'm a believer.

I laughed out loud about your feeling that you are the bad toy house. I feel like we are the *no* toy house. Just when I think,

"Oh, my God, Alex is so-o-o-o spoiled with all this stuff, it's a good thing she's too little to know it," I'll go over to someone else's house and feel instantly like Alex has no toys nor a full library like THIS family. I try to figure out if all their stuff is in one room, so it looks like a lot, instead of at our house, where there's stuff in virtually every room. (Something I swore I would not do as a pregnant woman.)

Okay, I am officially extremely tired. It's 9:00 p.m. Time to cut the grapes in half and peel the apple slices for tomorrow.

Zzzzzz, renee

From: amy krouse rosenthal <amy@suba.com>
To: "Renee Raab Whitcombe"

Dear Renee

While your home is on a truck somewhere between L.A. and Cleveland, and your life is in utter disarray, I distract you with this:

Day: Yesterday. Time: that 8:07 zone, where we're all running around like freaks, kids are eating cereal, I'm trying to brush Paris's hair while she's eating her maple-and-brown-sugar oatmeal, someone can't find a shoe, another mother calls to confirm a playdate after school, and I realize my breath really stinks.

So then Paris dropped her toast, and it broke in half. And if you look on that chart all mothers are handed as they leave the delivery room, and pan down to the bottom of page 2, you'll see that "broken toast or pretzel rod = 42 minutes of hysteria."

I wanted to call, "Do-over!"

Suddenly, I was acutely aware of my fantasy breakfast routine, and how far we are from achieving/living it. Here's what I have in my head: One day, I will be able to begin the day in a calm way. Our mornings will be slow and easy and full of beauty. The kids will glide into the kitchen and get their backpacks together without being prompted, while I scramble eggs with one hand and French braid Paris's hair with the other. The soundtrack to this little film? Mozart or Natalie Merchant. Oh, and yes, in this fantasy, I'm actually showered and dressed.

I recently toyed with the idea of making a documentary with a producer friend here about morning routines—only because I am dying to see how other families do it. Jason keeps telling me that simply waking up before the kids would help solve a lot of the problem. But I do so love to sleep. Will you please be a good friend and tell me that your mornings are worse than mine?

Love,

amy

From: "Renee Raab Whitcombe"
To: amy krouse rosenthal <amy@suba.com>

Renee Whitcombe wrote:

Amy,

We've been here exactly one week. Wow, what a week it's been. My journey out here started with sitting on the runway in Newark for 4 hours before finally taking off for the 1-hour flight. After staying with my folks last week, I was thinking on the plane about writing an article called something like "How to Survive Being a Guest with Your Toddler in an Unbabyproofed Home." The little subtopics would be "Showering," "Cleaning Up—How Little Is Still Polite?", "Diaper Disposal—From Tricky to Honest," "Rules for Climbing and Jumping," "Short-Term Insurance Options," and of course a special section on how to get pasta out from between the keys of a piano.

Let me respond to your e-mail more directly at this point. I can't tell you my mornings are as crazy as yours . . . yet. For starters, I have one-third the number of children, so the lack of consequences is exponential. Also, Alex is kind of a brunch girl. Not really interested in food until she's been up 2 to 3 hours.

But I do agree with Jason about getting up earlier than the kids, as painful as it may be. If I get up even a half-hour before Alex, get the bottle and snacks ready, put my walking clothes on, pack my day bag for later, and enter a few Quicken receipts, I can turn her around in no time. If I wait till I hear her to get out of bed and stagger in with a cold bottle still wearing my pajamas, I can't get us out the door in less than an hour-and-a-half. I don't know why this is true, but it's true every time. I wish there were some way of slapping myself to sleep early enough that doing this weren't such a hardship.

Of course, anything I am capable of now may be a joke after this kid comes on September 7.

R

From: amy krouse rosenthal <amy@suba.com>
To: "Renee Raab Whitcombe"

Renee

So there you are in Cleveland. Ah, Cleveland, the land of Cleve. (What is a cleve?) By now, I imagine you're settled, i.e., you have baking soda in the fridge.

I have to tell you this story, totally true, and a highlight since we last spoke.

Jason and I went to this new sushi restaurant in Bucktown. That night, they were serving an exotic delicacy—shots of electric baby eel! Intrigued and feeling brave, Jason ordered one. Intrigued and feeling like I would vomit, I watched as he downed a little glass of alive, green, squirmy things. This wasn't just an appetizer, Renee, it was an *event.*

Jason said he could feel a couple of the eels trying to shimmy back up his throat. Our mutual and immediate reaction to all this was: The kids would have LOVED to see this, particularly the boys, who were still talking about the chocolate-covered grasshoppers we brought home from a Mexican restaurant for them 3 years ago.

Sunday morning, we shared the big eel news with them. Justin was, as we suspected, blown away, captivated; he then proceeded to tell anyone who would listen the story of Daddy and the green eel. He would tell it with such detail and drama: "Okay, so there was a little glass, about so big . . ."

A couple days later, while driving home, I was thinking about it again, about how exciting this eel adventure was to the boys, how in awe they were, how impressed and proud of their Dad they were, how much I loved watching Justin tell the story . . . I looked up and the license plate of the car in front of me was: eel 48.

Sometimes the world nods along with you.

Other highlights:

—Finding a dismantled swingset in the alley and hauling the slide over to our backyard.

—Having all the kids on my lap the other morning, telling a story about a shark I think, it was divine, not the story, having them on my lap, even though one of them was smooshing my ankle and it was killing me.

—After 3 weeks of having storage boxes stacked up in my closet blocking half my drawers and thinking every day about taking them down to the basement, finally doing it. Such joy and satisfaction upon completion.

—And last, after spilling an entire box of linguine on the floor while making dinner, and being bummed, how stupid, what a waste, I realized, wait a second—cooking this food and sterilizing it to be clean is exactly one and the same. Saved. Excellent.

Love,

Amy

P.S. I can't remember anything anymore, can you? I open the cabinet and can't remember what I was about to get. I catch myself putting the sponge away in the fridge. I can no longer retain the names of my cousins. Which leads me to ask: Does trying to jog my memory count as exercise?

From: Renee Whitcombe
Sent: Fri, 23 Jun 2000 14:42:09 -0400
To: amy krouse rosenthal <amy@suba.com>
Subject: Do I HAVE to have one?

Hi Amy,

We are getting settled. Even my lavender master bedroom does not seem so strange anymore. The baking soda is indeed in the fridge, and I have stopped using a city map every time I back out of the driveway. We have activities, music classes, swimming lessons, a play group, and even season passes to Sea World and the zoo. I would say we are officially starting to have fun.

I am surprising myself at how terrific this full-time mom thing is. I thought I'd be bored or somehow just not into the patience it requires. Instead, I feel like Alex and I are getting so close and so in sync at a time when she is truly a fascinating little creature. (Make that a fascinating creature who has six teeth coming in all at once.) Admittedly, I do need to take a break from being Mommy all the time and find a way to be Renee sometimes too. And I don't just mean during her nap, when what I am doing is laundry, restocking diaper bags, and making bite-size snacks. But until we find the right person and the right recipe, it's working fine and I am really grateful that I am having this experience.

This pregnancy is not as fun as the last one. For one thing, I already look like I did the day before I delivered Alex. Also, I feel older this time. I refuse to indulge that fact, but at the end of the day, I am just trashed. This old bod probably should have started doing this at 30 instead of 36. I am entirely conscious of my surging hormones, too.

Thank you for offering up that loss-of-memory trait. I am getting sincerely scared of having a second child because I don't think my personal Alzheimer's could go to another level, but what if it does? That's the limbo that I fear. These early stages, where at least you know that it's happening, are one thing, but then the degrees of it all get more serious (and perhaps more blissful?). What if I think I just fed the baby and it's been like 11 hours? What if I forget to take the baby off my breast for 11 straight hours? What if I find myself stuffing hamburger meat into the ignition of my car while my keys sit quietly by the ice-cube trays? What if Alex asks me where Mom is? Will I know?

Renee ■

insight

A Mother's Heroes

My "heroes" vary with my state of mind/phases of the moon. But here is a collection of women who have inspired me over the years and who, except for one, happen to go by the name Ann(e). (Quickly glance at the word "Heroes" . . . did you see the word "Oreos," too?)

ANNE MORROW LINDBERGH, ANNE SEXTON, ANNE LAMOTT, and ANNE FRANK

Writers

AYN RAND

Writer (*I am woman, hear me Roark.*)

ANN KROUSE

A woman I know who raised four children, ran and grew a business with her husband, can still, to this day, tell you which dress her daughter wore to the Turnabout dance, never put the ketchup bottle on the table, was organized—she still has the receipt, 35 years later, in a well-marked file, to her children's baby furniture—and somehow made each of her children feel like they were her favorite.

ANN B. DAVIS

Proof you can really make do with one outfit.

GINA

My neighbor, because at a neighborhood store, I watched as her kids sat quiet and motionless in their chairs for 20 minutes while she shopped.

lesson five

Magic Wand

TRADING IN THE OLD YOU

Let's say you . . . what should we make it? . . . got the big promotion? . . . wrote a screenplay? . . . wrote a book? Let's make it a book, why not?

And that book took you roughly forever to write. And then 50 rejection letters later, it finally finds a publisher. And a year after that, it comes out. And it's like the biggest thing in your entire life . . . and . . . and . . . and guess what? The world does not stop. Silly you, you imagined that the world *would* stop. You imagined that all the bookstore owners would call you and say, "We just got your book. We're getting rid of all the other books and are just carrying yours!" You imagined that hordes of old friends and colleagues would call and say, "I'm so sorry we fell out of touch. I didn't realize you were so . . . relevant. Can you come over for tea?" You imagined that all your problems and idiosyncrasies would disappear, and that each and every day you would wake up looking fabulous, vibrant, airbrushed.

In other words, you imagined that the the old you would be traded in for a new, shiny, leather-interior you.

***

When I got engaged, my mother took me shopping for what was once upon a time called a *trousseau*, a gift of garments mothers traditionally sent their virgin daughters off with as they began their new lives as wives. It was totally sweet and old-fashioned and unnecessary and so my mom. It was there in the lingerie department that she held up these lacy, shoulder-padded, undershirt things, and said, "You will definitely need a couple of these." I had never worn—let alone seen—a lacy shoulder-padded undershirt thing before. But I figured 1) my mom knew what she was doing, and 2) when I got married, perhaps minutes after exchanging vows—*poof!* I would be a different person. I couldn't quite picture who that different person was, but I vaguely imagined that the married Amy would be more grown up, more organized, more . . . *better*. Basically, that I would suddenly have a pressing need for lacy, shoulder-padded undershirt things.

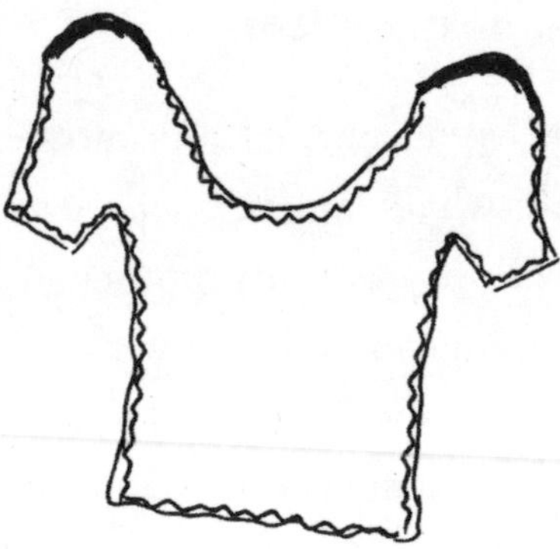

After 7 years of marriage, and 7 years of looking at the undershirt things with the tags still on, I finally put them in a bag to be donated. It was kinda sad, but also a relief—I no longer had to sit around wondering when my glamourous genes were going to kick in. My predominant genes seem to be of the ripped-denim variety.

Admittedly, before I leave this model-infested Earth, I would like, for just one day, to trade driveways for runways. It would be great to strut, to sway, to *match*. But, alas, for now, my designer of choice is DKNWhy Bother.

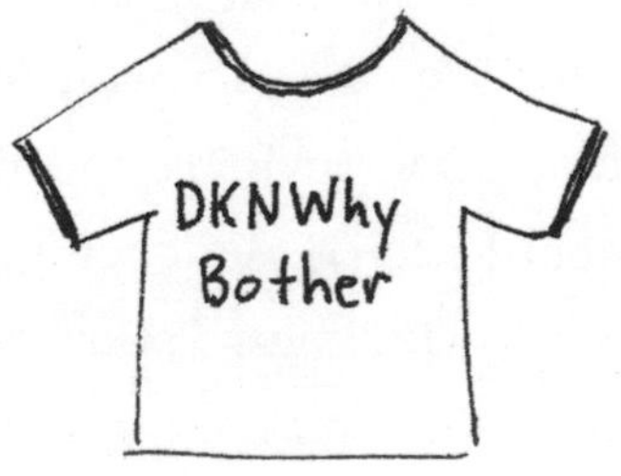

***

Somewhere along the way my boys got it in their heads that what we needed around the house was a magic wand—"a *real* magic wand, Mom"—so

> Right here... right now... please promise me that you'll never chat on your cell phone while walking your child into school.

we went to the costume store and asked to see their magic wand inventory. We eventually settled on one that looked especially sparkly and authentic. The boys waited eargerly as I paid for it, and debated what they would become first—tigers? cheetahs? freak mutant lizards? I didn't know how I was going to get through this episode—I was already feeling nauseated anticipating their inevitable and massive disappointment—but I played along with it and hoped that playing along with it was a good idea in the first place. I unwrapped the plastic and said, "Okay, let's do it." There they stood, 60 pounds (combined) of pure faith and excitement.

"Abracadabra, turn Justin and Miles into tigers!" They looked at each other. Nope. Still boys. I tried again, a bit louder. "Abracadabra, TURN JUSTIN AND MILES INTO TIGERS!" Even years later, I still haven't found a way to accurately convey to you just how desperately I wanted a miracle to occur that afternoon. A miracle of biblical, or at least of Jenny Jones, proportions. Of course you know the rest: no poofs of smoke, no disappearing boys, no jungle escapades.

***

To this day, the boys frequently ask me—and they are completely sincere in this—"Mom, when you finally get your real magic wand, will you change us into ______________?"

And I promise them, "Yes, when I get a real magic wand, *if* I can ever find a real magic wand, I will be happy to change you into a __________." And I mean it, I so very much mean it, and I wish I could, because I would. Somehow the mere possibility of it all satisfies them for the time being, and they proceed to talk about what life will be like when they are __________. They will be able to jump higher, run faster, and not wear a coat!

It would be easy to dismiss this as simply an

example of the active imaginations of children. *A boy one minute, and a tiger the next, Ha, ha, isn't that sweet?* Adults aren't all that different when it comes to transformation fantasies. We're just less direct about it. They openly want to be tigers; we secretly want to be Tiger Woods, or at least have his swing.

***

If you sat me down, took me by the hands, and asked, "Amy, do you really think that when you go to get your haircut, you will walk out of the salon a taller, thinner, more likable person?" I'd have to answer, "Uh, yeah." I'm hoping that's okay. I'm hoping the therapists out there are nodding their heads, going, "Ah, yes, that's a classic example of, wait, it's right here on page 29, yes, Unrealistic Transformation Delusion—totally common, fairly normal."

I refuse to accept that even if I get the haircut, the book deal, the tiger stripes and tail, that I'm still going to be the same bundle of skin and bones and neurons. That I'm still going to have the same fingerprints, blood type, and four-digit cash machine code. That I'm still going to have the same unorganized junk drawer in the kitchen.

I've tried time and again to ditch myself, cut myself off at the pass, but nothing seems to work. There I am, same as ever. I think all roads of self-analysis/chin-rubbing lead to the same realization, one that was summed up nicely in this aphorism: *Wherever you go, there you are.* Which I guess in the end, is okay with me, because I don't know about you, but I could sure use the company. ■

mother wit

A Mother's Hidden Talents

Here's what's great about having kids. You can be really bad at something, but because they can't do that thing at all and perhaps have never even seen anybody do it, they think you are good at it. For example, I doodled this the other day:

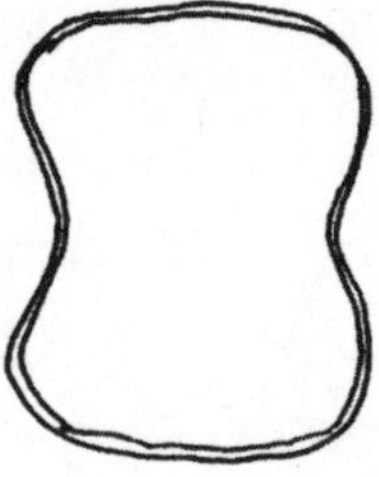

My son Justin says, "Wow, Mom, you draw really good toast!"

lesson six

Ruts, Frogs, and Jellybeans

ON GETTING UNSTUCK

When the boys were a little less than 2 and 3 plus, we moved them into the same room because we wanted bedtime to be a nightmare, I mean, because we needed to get the other bedroom ready for the baby who'd be arriving soon.

For weeks—I won't say how many—bedtime was an ordeal. We tried to stick to our same routine—after all, it had served us well for so long—but it didn't seem to hold the weight of two small boys. But we: kept at it. We: held our ground. We: plugged away. We let them cry at the top of the stairs, let them wail for more water. We took away dessert, took away movies, took away their college funds. Wedidn'tbudge. We kept hoping that if we did it this way long enough, they would see that we *meant it*, our point would finally settle in.

It didn't, they didn't. It got to the point where I would become queasy every evening anticipating the frustration and anxiety that lay ahead, another hour's worth of evidence in the argument against my competence as a mother.

> **Exhibit A:** The Rosenthals' 19-year-old au pair, Chris, had no problem getting the boys to nap every afternoon. In awe, Amy would drill Chris daily for tactics—Did you keep their door open or closed? What were your exact words as you left the room? Were your arms dangling or folded when you spoke?

Then one morning, with the rare advantage of a sunny sky, clear mind, and clean sink, I had a *McEpiphany*. I realized that I was hitting my head against the same paint-chipped wall every night, which is so stupid when you consider the fact that we have a good 10 to 20 other paint-chipped walls in our house. We were in a rut.

I believe what happens with a rut is that you have to sink to the very bottom of it before you even realize that you are in it. If you're only a little bit into a rut, you can still see a sliver of light above you. But when you're deep in the rut, it's superdark, the oxygen level drops, you can't see, you have trouble breathing, and you realize, oh boy, I'm in a big fat rut, and you have no choice but to make a mad dash for the nearest exit.

In that instant, I knew exactly what I had to do; it was so obvious, so simple. I grabbed a piece of paper and a pen and called my boys over. "Tell me everything you need at night in order to go to sleep. This is going to be your list, your ideas."

"Stories."

I drew a book.

"Water."

I drew a glass of water.

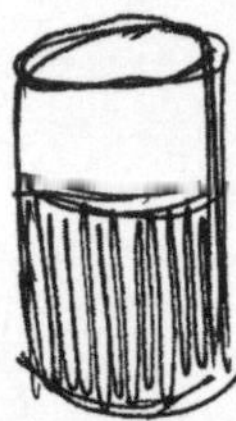

"Paper and pen." (They liked to fall asleep "writing" in bed.)

I drew a piece of paper and a pen.

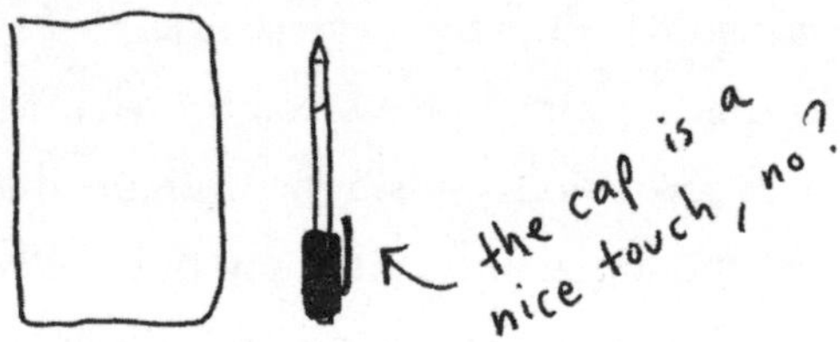
the cap is a
nice touch, no?

"A kiss goodnight."

I drew lips.

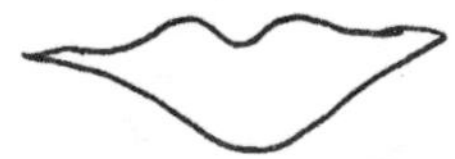

We had our list, or rather we had *their* list. While this was pretty much (i.e., exactly) what we had been providing for them each night, the difference was that in a nonbedtime, nonconfrontational moment, they were given the opportunity to tell me what they wanted and needed, and I listened, I just listened, no exaggerated exhaling, just plain, easy FM listening. Their thoughts were translated into something tangible that they could own and look at. They were pleased and proud.

I walked the chart upstairs, taped it to their door, and at bedtime 6 hours later, had them tell me what we were to do first, had them walk me through the ritual. *What comes after water again?* I gave them their pen and paper, their kisses goodnight, and closed the door. And that was that.

***

"Synopsis of Rut #2:" Dinnertime is totally chaotic. Kids getting up and down. Conversation consists of "*Now* can I have dessert? How many bites do I have to eat?" Keep trying. Chaos prevails. Keep trying. Chaos prevails. Recognition of rut. Sit down one Sunday morning. Ask them how many

> Cool tip: Put a mini marshmallow in the bottom of the sugar cone to prevent the ice cream from dripping.

minutes is fair to sit in seat and eat dinner. 20. 11. One hundred eighty-eleven. We take the average. 14 minutes. We will put a timer on table, so no need to ask how many bites since everyone knows timer going off = dessert time. Sunday night. Put timer on table. Actual eating and sitting and conversing. Timer goes off. They get dessert. 14-minute rule a hit. Epilogue. Occasionally, kids even ask us to set back timer, want to eat and talk more.

***

Throwing a rut under the microscope, we can see two distinct strains: There's the Conflict Rut, such as the ones described above. The thing with Conflict Ruts—and I seem to continually forget and relearn this—is that it's always just a *slight* shift of the dial that will get me back on course. Instead of digging myself deeper and deeper into the same hole, I put down the shovel, move 2 inches to the left, and there's the answer.

Then there's the Boredom Rut, a different beast entirely, known for attacking clear skies and leaving the unsuspecting victim in a fog of ugh 'n' ennui. One minute you're doing just fine, thriving on your daily domestic routine, and then—*boom!*—the kids are grumpy, and you feel like dyeing your hair. I find that there's a tricky balance for me between knowing when to be consistent/honoring thy routines (which the kids do thrive on) and when to incite mini, antiboredom revolutions. Oscar Wilde said, "Consistency is the last refuge of the unimaginative." Granted, he was childless, not to mention the best partygirl in town; nonetheless, this sentiment has flittered in and out of my consciousness throughout my mothering years, resurfacing and empowering me when I needed it most.

***

My absolute favorite book as a child was *Jellybeans for Breakfast.** Do you know it? I don't remember the whole story, but it was basically what you'd gather from the title: A little girl is delighted to find one morning that jellybeans are being served. Jellybeans! Now this did not require a lot of money or planning on her parents' part—I mean, the bag of jellybeans cost what? $1.29—but the impact it had on the character (and us spectators) was huge. Sick of the morning routine and the same three cereals in rotation, I suspect the mom did this as much for herself as she did for her daughter. With bathrobe and jellybean bag, this mom marched into battle against the Rut and emerged victorious. Oh, I can still see that page with all the jellybeans—beautiful bright yellow, orange, red, green, purple jelly beans. I was so excited for her.

---

*I have tried to find this book again, spoken with out-of-print book searching companies, each attempt in vain. If you can lead me to a copy of this book, I will send your child a year's worth of jellybeans, in the form of monthly care packages. Promise. E-mail me at amy@suba.com.

***

Not too long ago, I read about a 15-pound ceramic lawn-frog ornament that was stolen from the yard of John and Gertrude Knight, a couple in Massachusetts. About 10 days after the frognapping, the Knights received a letter that said, "Tired of sitting on the lawn. Love, the Frog." Over the next few months, the couple received letters from the frog from more than 20 countries, along with photos of him in various international locales (an Amsterdam café, on a gondola in Venice, on a newspaper box in Honolulu). About 8 months after the frog's mysterious departure, a white limo pulled up with the frog seatbelted in the backseat. The couple never found out who was behind the craziness (the driver was hired by an anonymous "Mr. Frog").

This frog has become my hero. I think of him, supposedly doomed to a life of lawn-sitting, and remind myself: If an amphibian *tchatchke* can manage to free itself of a rut, surely I should be able to manage. ■

A Rhyming Summary of the Universe

It is a bit of a challenge to eat steak with a spoon.

Don't show up at 20 after if you agreed to 12 noon.

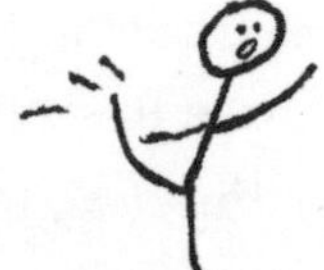

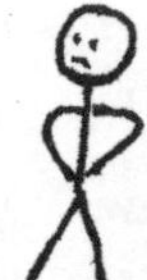

Mt. Rushmore's not in Russia, though they do sound alike.

You'll fall roughly 68 times when you first ride your bike.

You might be your least charming when it matters the most.

Really, it is not a tragedy when you burn a piece of toast.

Don't pretend to get it if you've no clue what they're talking about.

Choose the small room with the window over the big one without.

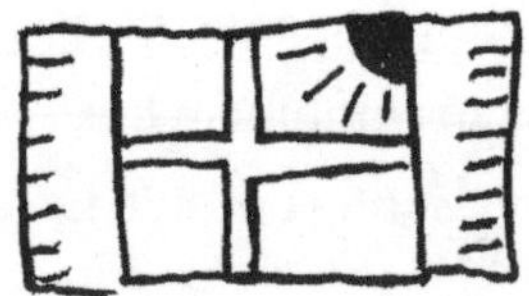

Please don't expect someone else to unmake your mess.
When offered seconds at a dinner party say, "Why, thank you, yes."
Ask not, "What will you give me if I help with the dishes?"
Give away two—okay, one—if you're granted three wishes.

Do the worst part of your homework first instead of saving it for later.
Stand up for your brother, sister, or some picked-on first grader.

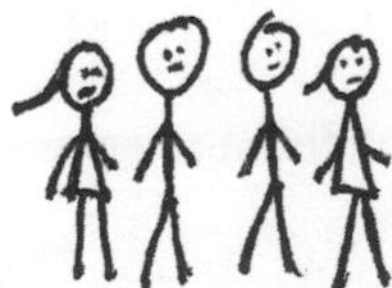

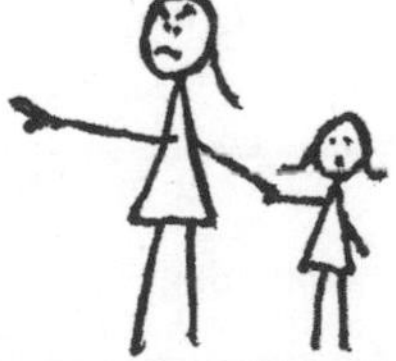

Go and jump in the puddle—just bring an extra pair of socks.
Think twice before flocking to where everyone else flocks.

Hang on to your old friends while making ones that are
different and newer.
Some days your zipper will jam and your ice cream will fall
down a sewer.

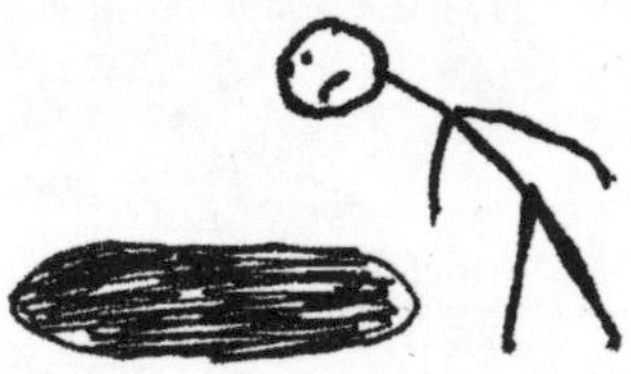

Raise your hand if you know the answer, keep it down if
you don't.
It's hard to climb to the top with "can'ts," "nos," and
"won'ts."

Despite your best efforts, your goldfish may stop
swimming.
It is most unattractive to always be gimme, gimme,
gimme-ing.

If your neighbor is sick, cheer him up with Hershey's kisses and soup.

Cursive takes some practice with all those

~~fancy twirl~~

~~fancy twirls and loop~~

fancy twirls and loops.

No matter how big the cake, there are always only four corner pieces.

Uncles, by trade, steal noses from their nephews and nieces.

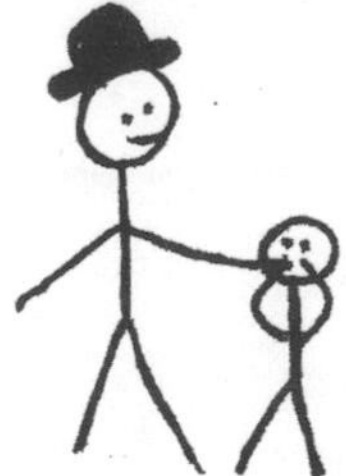

Learn how to listen. (Did you hear what I just said?)
When you roll a 5, don't sneak 6 spaces ahead.
Your parents will often annoy you for no certain reason.
Enjoy blueberries while you can (they have a very short season).

64 crayons you do not really need.
To be happy with 3 is to be happy indeed.

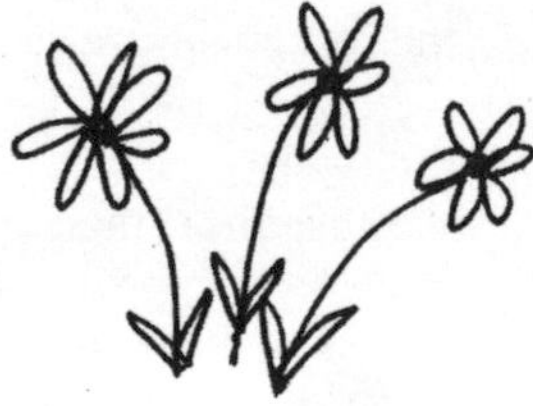

lesson seven

Snapshots from My Guilt Trip

NO MATTER WHAT YOU FORGET TO PACK, IT ALL WORKS OUT IN THE END

Though they originally intended to go back to work, one by one I watched my friends and acquaintances quit their jobs to stay home and be with their child(ren). Any discussion about work and children ultimately led to the same refrain: *Work means nothing to me now/oh, baby, oh/I couldn't stand being away from my baby all day/oh, baby, oh. . . .*

Shouldn't I be part of this chorus, or at least singing backup? What's wrong with me that I don't want to quit my job? I'm lucky enough to be able to conceivably *not* work. I have a choice here, and I'm choosing not to not work?

What kind of mother am I? I've just had a baby, for God's sake. We're not talking about a new goldfish or a new couch, but a *baby*! Our miracle Love Child!

I'm fairly certain that I am not the only woman who has continued to work after having kids. But at the time, those first couple of months after Justin was born, all I seemed to hear was that every (good) new mom was staying home. That's the info I was tuning in to, the only message that was coming in clearly, like when you cut your waist-length hair and you hate it, and no matter where you go, all you see, all you *notice*, are women with

L

O

N

G

uncut hair.

Something like that.

So the wind flipped the pages of the calendar . . . February . . . March . . . April . . . and in the course of just plowing through the days and nights (though who could tell the difference then?), I gradually became more and more comfortable in my new mother skin. The dark, jagged Guilt faded to a soft, lowercase g kind of guilt, and I somehow came to terms with the fact that working was just part of my deal, and that having 1 baby or 10 babies probably wouldn't change that. It was a notation on my chart that I could lie about but never really alter.

And whew, was it a good thing I got over that guilt, because I needed to make room for a whole other slew of issues I was going to feel guilty about in the weeks and years ahead.

Guilty that I wasn't filling out the baby book properly. Guilty that I stopped breastfeeding at 3 months, then with the next, guilty I stopped breastfeeding at 9 months, then with the next, guilty I stopped breastfeeding at 14 months. Guilty that I wasn't making homemade baby food, and then when I started making homemade baby food,

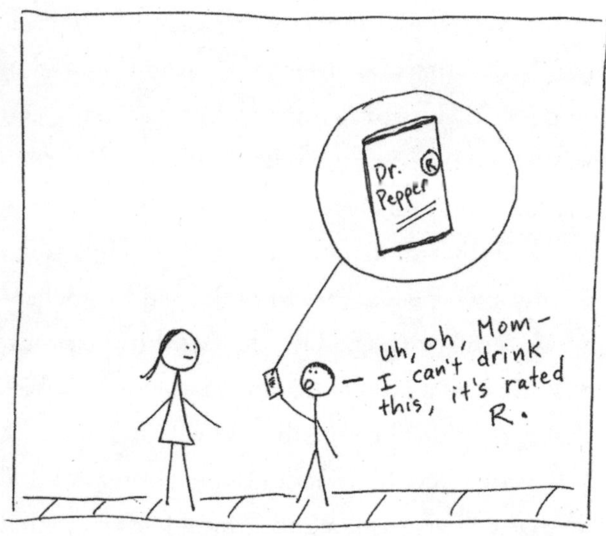
Dr. Pepper ®
Uh, oh, Mom—
I can't drink
this, it's rated
R.

guilty that I would serve the homemade baby food with a side of Burger King fries. Guilty that we weren't videotaping the kids every Sunday. Guilty that I didn't make it a habit to cover them with Johnson's Baby Lotion after each bath. Guilty that I didn't make a homemade cowboy/Batman/M&M costume for Halloween. Guilty that I didn't sign the kids up for enough after-school activities or guilty that I signed them up for too many or not the right ones. Guilty that I didn't really want to listen to that whole long story about—I don't even know what it was about, something involving recess and a *Tyrannosaurus rex* and Ethan Bresler. Guilty that I had packed Goldfish for snacks when the mom next to me whipped out a Tupperware container full of garbanzo beans and soy cheese. Guilty that I didn't wait until they were 17 to introduce sugar into their diets.

The upside to guilt is that it acts as a mental flashlight—illuminating a moment or situation that might have otherwise slipped into my subconscious unexamined. So I take that guilt and all its condiments—insecurity, doubt, shame—place it on a lazy Susan, and look at it from every angle. Then and only then am I able to assess if I'm feeling guilty because I do in fact feel the need to alter something (yes, I need to follow through on the music lessons), or if the guilt was actually a trapdoor that when passed through led me to a place of heightened certainty and confidence (yes, I *am* okay with being a working mom and I *am* pro-Goldfish).

***

I had a blessed childhood—daily doses of love, encouragement, dinner rolls. But I don't remember every day, every meal, every heart-to-heart. I don't think we retain our childhood in large, clear, decade-long chunks; I think we remember in flashes, in nuances, in general gists. Images rise and fall in my consciousness: the red scratchy carpet in the family room and how it felt on my elbows while I lay with my head propped up on my fists and watched *The Carol Burnett Show* with my sister; the smell of onions sautéed in butter, and my dad dipping white bread into it; the way my room seemed so new and fresh and fun when I rearranged the furniture; going to the shoe store with my mom, examining each contender, leaving with the one perfect pair of school shoes, the pair that best represented me; the song my mom sang to me every time she had to take my temperature; gulping apple juice straight from the jar in the front seat of the Jeep on the way home from a tennis match, my dad driving; hanging out in the kitchen with my friends, eating, always eating; my best friend Rosalie's driveway, so steep; how my dad never knew where we kept the forks.

> My pal M. C. told me that her dad, out of nowhere, apologized for not letting her and her sister ride the ferris wheel at that one beach they went to . . . 30 years ago! She had remembered those summer beach vacations as sweet and lovely and perfect; and there's her pop, still agonizing.

That's what we're creating for our children—not a single full-length film, but dozens of 30-second unrelated shorts. I'm hoping that if Jason and I can strive to create an arena where they generally feel recognized, appreciated, loved, and disciplined, we can be pretty sure that, by and large, the good feelings and memories will prevail. Not to say that we can skip town for a few years—oh, they'll never remember this anyway—but missing a t-ball game or forgetting to put the dollar under the pillow one night* will be a mere blip on the radar screen.

To what degree my own parents felt guilty about not doing this, or doing that, I can't say exactly, but I would guess it wasn't much; they were pretty confident in their choices and parenting style. (I'm sure my dad would be *more* than happy to tell you what he knows about parenting. E-mail him at paulk@honoring.com) But what a waste of time if they had spent countless hours feeling guilty, when in the end, what I absorbed, what I now remember, is that my childhood felt really, really good. ■

---

*It took me a week to get over the guilt of forgetting to put the dollar under Justin's pillow, even though we saved ourselves: We were on vacation at the time, and we told him the Tooth Fairy had trouble finding him in this foreign house, so (sneak, run, hide it) she must have left it by the front door. And lo and behold, there it was by the front door.

mother wit

Waiting in Line for My Teenagers

A CAMEO BY BARB COOKE

My first brush with being irrelevant happened 6 years ago when we were late for a dentist appointment and couldn't find my 7-year-old daughter. I finally found Jenny in the cold, dark garage. In the car. In the front passenger seat. My sons were aghast. "Get out of that seat! I ride shotgun today!" yelled 14-year-old Ben, grabbing her arm and trying to wrench her out the car door. She braced her feet against the dashboard, latched onto the steering wheel, and squealed, "It's my turn to sit in the front next to Mommy!"

Twelve-year-old Jon stared at her incredulously, then bellowed, "You don't even know how to turn on the radio!" Then he spat out the worst insult he could hurl. "The only reason you want to sit up front is because you *love* Mom! How stupid is that?"

As the mother of teens, I suddenly found myself on the periphery instead of center stage in their harried lives. Being smothered with hugs and kisses and cries of "Mommy! I need you now!" screeched to a halt with puberty and morphed into "Mom! I need these shirts, jeans, shoes, and this CD burner now!" I shuffled uncertainly to the back of the line to wait for those hugs and kisses as the line continually swelled with boyfriends, girlfriends, and best friends.

But we parents of teens are like chameleons, quick-change artists who adapt in a millisecond. I learned that I could disguise myself, and they would need me again. I doffed my chauffeur's cap and reported on call 24/7 to ferry them to school and friends' houses and shopping malls and concerts. They never guessed it was me posing as an ATM machine that received no deposits but always spewed out money for allowance, dances, gifts, cars, clothes, tutors, and tuition.

Bet they'd be shocked to know that it was me dressed as Fifi the maid when I stood by my post at the washer and dryer each day, dutifully turning their shirts right side out and matching all those socks, never flinching at the odor of their gym clothes that were so stiff they stood up by themselves but were only being washed because "Our gym teacher made all of us take our stuff home or we're not getting our report cards."

I was a disaster-relief worker the day I ventured into Ben's room and stared in disbelief at the scene on his floor. Lopsided piles of clean clothes lent an interesting topographical touch. Tennis ball cans and damp towels covered his bed, while his comforter dangled sideways to the floor. Bowls with 3-day-old congealed milk and petrified cereal crowded his desk, spoons embedded in the thick goop. I only gagged once.

My multiple hats masked me as their number one fan who baked in the sun at Ben's tennis matches, bundled up in the whipping wind at Jon's football games, clapped at Jenny's plays. I played the somber policeman when they came in late, talked back, or skipped school. And I was Academy Award–winning material as the patient in the intensive care unit, admitted for being deathly sick with worry (about them fighting with strangers, getting shot, overdosing on drugs or alcohol, sexual assault, getting cut from the team, not making the right friends, getting pregnant or getting AIDS, a good grade point average, a good future).

But each night, as I slipped out of my disguises and stared at my naked face in the mirror, I wondered if my three teenagers would ever understand why I did the things I did and said the things I said. Would they ever know how much I really love them?

Then, on one of the many days when Ben and I were screaming at each other about how ungrateful and selfish he was, and how he wished he lived with any other family in the world, he heaved his backpack to the floor in disgust and slammed the door in my face. That was when I saw his English paper, the one titled "My Rock," the one my rebellious, defiant son wrote about the day he came home and found out I had to have surgery:

> *Now the worry became pure, unadulterated fear. What would I do without my mom? Okay, I admit, sometimes I acted like I'd be happier without the nagging and complaining and every other annoying mother*

quality, but those aspects of our relationship vanished at that moment. I could only think of the loving, nurturing mom who would do anything for me and my brother and sister. She was the rudder on my ship, steering me through the stormy seas of childhood. She was my rock. Although I was 16, I felt like a small child again, reliant upon my mother for everything. I would be lost without her.

And here I am back at the front of the line again.

Stop.
Drop everything.
Dad has a cold.

lesson eight

Life Sentence

A STREAM OF THE UNCONSCIONABLE

Today, when I was picking up my dry cleaning, the owner said, wait, before you go, this envelope, we found $10 in your pocket last week, a white envelope with a few words in blue ink, "Rosenthal, $10, from the pocket on shirt, March 6, 2000",

such a gesture, finding this money, money he could have so easily taken, we would have never known if he had, putting it in a special envelope, such a pure, kind gesture, startling in the midst of all our bad news lately, one piece of new, bad information after another, the processing of each new piece, making the necessary phone calls, thinking about the new information, wondering, it's so tiring, the wondering and the processing,

and so this gesture, he stopped whatever it was he was doing, put down whatever was in his hand so he could go find an envelope and a pen to make a note, this gesture in the midst of our babysitter leaving and the flood in our basement and my father having angioplasty,

and my mother-in-law getting a black eye from a swinging camera, so silly, nothing really, but an example, fine to not fine in one-half of 1 second . . .

then out of nowhere, something so tragic and awful, worst of all, I'm sorry to have even mentioned the babysitter and the flood, they mean nothing, this means everything, it is so real, and it happened, it's happening to these parents right now, their child, gone, there one moment, laughing and walking and spilling things, and then gone,

the parents, I can't stop thinking about the parents, how will they move on, how will they ever eat anything more than toast, a loss that will swallow them up, a loss that may send them to India, they can't go to the movies, they can't run out for sushi, the only thing that makes sense is going to India,

and my husband is on the way to this boy's funeral, we were away for the weekend when we heard the news, so he had to take a train back to the city, the rest of us would come home later in the day in the minivan, and then my husband calls from home, hi, I'm home, guess how I got in the door? and I think, our house was broken into, of course, we were robbed while we were away, but that's good, we should be robbed, it's exactly right, that should absolutely happen at a time like this, I'm glad they stole the CD player, some spoons, some jewelry I don't wear anyway, why don't I care about jewelry, women are supposed to care about jewelry,

but it's not that, we weren't robbed, he got into the house because he took the keys, my keys, the keys with the minivan key on it, there he is in Chicago with the key, and here we are in Michigan with the minivan but no key to drive it back, how will we get home? my husband will have to drive our other car all the way back to

Michigan and give us the key, he will miss the funeral, his leaving at the crack of dawn to take the train will have been in vain, that rhymes: train/in vain, this can't rhyme, a child has died, nothing can ever rhyme again, my husband has to go to the funeral, he must go, there has to be another solution, yes, we will all go home in my in-laws' car, all seven of us in a car for four, that makes sense, we should be uncomfortable for the drive home, more than that certainly, but it's a start, we shouldn't have any leg room in light of what's happened,

we'll call you right back, we're going to see if we can all fit in the car, we're going to do a test run, and we put down the phone and we all get in the car, you sit on my lap, you two in the front, the rest of us in back, this will work, it's tight but it will work, we call back, you go to the funeral, we'll all drive home with your folks and we'll meet you back at the house midafternoon to get ready for the birthday party,

a birthday party, yes, our daughter's third birthday party, with balloons and wrapping paper and being happy and alive and asking for more frosting, a birthday party, after this funeral, have you ever? of course there's the issue of how and when will we get the minivan back home, we'll figure that out later, that minivan can sit there for a year for all I care, and my dad's heart, and the dead child, and the flooded basement, my whole house should fill up with water right now if there were any justice in the world everyone's house should flood out of respect for the dead child,

and still the envelope stopped me, comforted me, that's the way it is, a small white envelope, so kind, he wrote our name on it, to be sure to give it to us, "from the pocket on shirt." ■

insight

The Music of Motherhood

Here are some of the best sounds in the world; sounds that remind you why you wanted to become a mom so badly in the first place. Next time you're online, you can click on www.mommymommy.com to actually hear these sounds.

SLURPING CEREAL

The kids are at the kitchen counter perched on their wooden stools, one, two, three children in a row, all hunched over their bowls, crunching and slurping Cinnamon Life.

"MOMMY'S HOME! MOMMY'S HOME!"

Who else but your children and that one psycho ex-boyfriend would put down whatever they're doing, run with flailing, ecstatic arms, and then gaze at you as if you were the Tooth Fairy, Good Humor Man, and the Messiah all wrapped in one, simply because a door opened and you were on the other side of it?

THE CRINKLING OF A DIAPER AS A TODDLER WALKS

To hear this is to immediately feel compelled to squeeze their poofy, padded tushes and kiss their soft, fat faces.

THE "HAPPY BIRTHDAY" SONG

There your child is, with all her friends and family around her in front of a large, themed sheet cake. This is exactly like the photos you've looked at hundreds of times over the years of you making a wish at your 1st and 5th and 9th birthdays. But now it's your 1-year-old and then your 5-year-old and then your 9-year-old making a wish. You'd give up all your wishes to have her one wish come true, and everyone is clapping for your child's existence. And then just like that, the eye-welling, heart-swelling moment is over as a herd of little people begin shrieking for a piece with Barbie's head.

SILENCE

But a very particular kind of silence. It's the silence that occurs when you have had a full day with the kids, and everyone is finally sanitized and asleep in bed, and you are now just walking down the stairs to a startling quiet room, a couch, and the new *Entertainment Weekly*.

ANOTHER CHILD GREETING YOUR CHILD WITH GLEE

It seems somehow miraculous that your child can venture out into the world and, completely on his own, by his own doing, emerge with a friend in hand. It's so cool how that works. And hearing this friend shout your child's name, which is shorthand for "Oh, good! My friend has arrived! And I am happy to see him!" is superb.

"I LOVE YOU, MOM."

Mmmmmm.

lesson nine

6:30 P.M., Central Standard Time

HOW CHANGING OUR DINNER PLANS CHANGED OUR LIVES

Jason and I didn't start the family dinner routine until Justin was about 2. For the first couple of years, we . . . I don't know what we did. We stood at the kitchen counter, ordered in, or ate leftovers from what we'd ordered in the night before; this, while we talked in staccato half-sentences about our day/went through the mail/fed Justin homemade pureed sweet potatoes (I lie. It was Stouffer's spinach soufflé).

Then Miles was born. We officially became a

family, a foursome, a scene from the box of a board game, minus the matching casualwear. Something about this new arrangement begged for a reevaluation of the kitchen counter routine. Sit-down dinners were something we'd always—though we didn't realize it until now—wanted. So we packed up our salt and pepper shakers and moved from the kitchen counter to the dining room. Not that we suddenly became people *avec* class: We still used cheap paper napkins, and someone invariably came to the table naked. Yet there we were each night, same time, same (high) chairs.

After a few months of eating actual meals at an actual table and enjoying it, something happened, I can't remember exactly how, but something happened that I would have never predicted: We began having Friday night Shabbat dinners. As in celebrating the Sabbath. Lighting candles. Blessing the bread. Using a tablecloth.

To illustrate the point of what an odd leap this was, I must back up for a minute. Throughout my childhood, I was Jewish precisely 54 times a year: on Rosh Hashana, on Yom Kippur, and every Sunday night when we had Chinese food. I was not Bat Mitzvahed, though I did fulfill some of the required credits by spending the better part of seventh and eighth grades throwing my arms up in the air to the song "Shout!"

I never write down the order number when ordering from a catalog, even though I pretend to do so. When the salesperson asks, "Do you have a pen handy?" I say, "Yeah, okay, B-8803-042," repeating it back to her as I'm spongeing off the countertop.

So here we were, partaking in a ritual that goes back thousands of years. Our era may have concocted the Internet and adhesive sticker postage stamps, but kudos to those gentlemen who invented Shabbat. Here's the gist: Come sundown Friday, all work must cease. You must not only stop working but you must begin partying *at once.* You must stop worrying about being productive and prosperous, and instead focus on and be grateful for what you have, for what and who is before you. You must eat good food with good friends and family. You must drink—*L'chaim!*—if you are of proper age and healthy heart. Sex is strongly encouraged.

Yes, okay, where do I sign?

Like snowflakes and haircuts, no two Shabbats in our home are ever the same. Sometimes we have friends over, sometimes family, sometimes nobody. Some Shabbats are mellow, others chaotic. Sometimes the food is edible, sometimes I overseason with coriander. We've made good friends through the ritual, and we've shared the experience with people of all faiths. It was not long before we realized that these Shabbats were now the very center of our family life. No matter what happens during the week—and something always does happen—in the back of our minds, and I mean children and adults alike, we can count on this one thing, this one constant, this one pretty hill perched somewhere just beyond Thursday.

Rosenthal Family's Shabbat Soy-Honey So-Easy Dressing

Whisk together:

- $\frac{1}{2}$ cup canola oil
- 3 tablespoons Kikkoman soy sauce
- 1 tablespoon honey

Serves 6.

The dining room table where all our sundry dinners and Shabbats occur has its own special role. The base of it is an old machine relic, some sort of iron braiding contraption we found at an antique artifacts shop. It's not the most practical item in our home (to wit: the glass top needs Windexing after every use), but it has a presence, a weight, an air of *I'm not going anywhere.* And so there it is, an anchor, not just for the thick sheet of glass, but, I hope, for the five people who break bread around it. ■

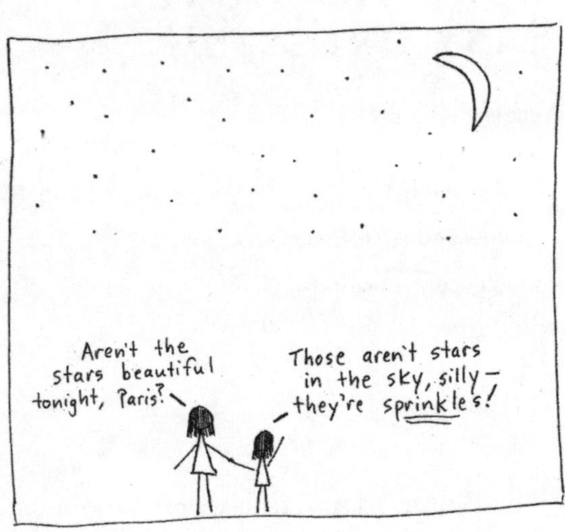
Aren't the stars beautiful tonight, Paris?
Those aren't stars in the sky, silly—they're sprinkles!

mother wit

The Cherry Falls from the Tree

A CAMEO BY DANIEL SPATUCCI

My brother, sister, and I were playing together one day as my parents got dressed for a rare dinner out. My father looked sharp in his best shirt and shiny silk tie—a lot different than he did when he left early each morning to drive his truck. He was freshly combed and coiffed when he became the victim of a vicious practical joke. It seems the jokester's incredibly clever idea was to fill the bathroom glass with water, so that when it was lifted, the water would spill all over the jokee.

Now wearing a sopping wet dress shirt and shiny silk tie, my father was intent on discovering the genius responsible for his predicament. He resorted to the time-honored technique of screaming, "Who did this?" Well, the jokester was ready and responded quickly, "Not me!" The jokester's sister caught on fast and echoed the denial. But the jokester's little brother was not fast enough and got both the blame and a sharp whack on his behind to help speed up his responses in the future.

Many years later, we were all enjoying one of the rare times that the whole family was together and started to tell all of the old family stories, mostly because our own kids now got a kick out of them. Something made me think of the water incident, so I asked if anyone remembered it, and to my surprise, no one did! Even my telling the story didn't jog anyone's memory, although it did get some laughs. I couldn't get over the fact that I'd carried this little guilt around for all those years, and no one else even remembered the incident.

My only reasonable course of action at this point was to shove this lesson down my kids' throats. When the laughs died down, I told them that maybe now they could see why it is better to tell the truth and take the punishment than to load themselves with the weight of the little guilts that accumulate over the years. My father had released his anger and went about changing his shirt and tie. My brother took the whack and forgot about it. I joked and lied and felt the guilt for 30 years.

One day last week, I came home to see that the lamppost on the front lawn was broken, clearly the act of a young person with not enough chores to keep him busy. Obeying the ancient instinct, I ran inside and screamed, "Who did this?"

The kids looked at each other, and from out of nowhere, the small voice of my 7-year-old whimpered, "I'm sorry, Dad, I did it."

Whatever anger was inside me instantly left, and I knelt down and gave him a big hug.

lesson ten

Scotch Tape on the Ukulele

WELCOME TO SELF-IMPORTANCE

A child loves his play, not because it's easy, but because it's hard.

—Benjamin Spock, *Baby and Child Care*

The Scotch tape epiphany didn't hit me until recently, but looking back, I realize it was on low simmer for the past 4 to 5 years. When Justin was 3, he had a little toy ukulele (now long broken and gone) and decided one afternoon that it was imperative that he cover the entire instrument with tape.

He was sitting there at the kitchen counter, so intently, with such devotion, putting tiny little pieces of tape all over the guitar. I completely remember thinking how pointless, what a waste of time, and, more important, what a waste of tape. I, for my part, was immersed in some list-making task; I dismissed his activity as insignificant and deemed mine significant. How lame is that?

Then, just last week (that would be the week of January 27, 2000), 2-year-old Paris put a piece of ribbon on the dining room floor and proceeded to tape it down in meticulous fashion. Not just one piece of tape or two. But piece after piece after piece, in a row, like railroad tracks, like this:

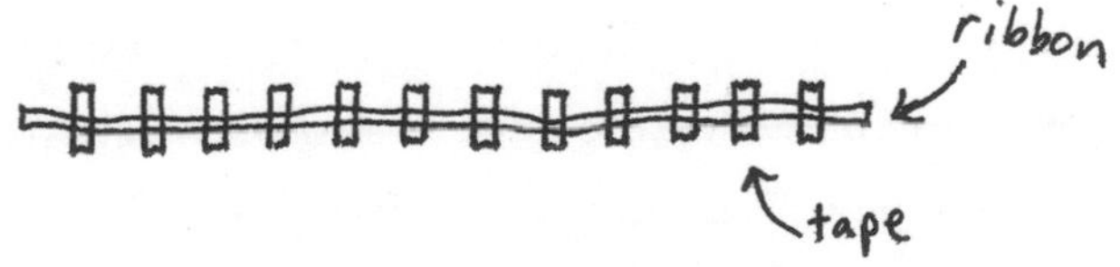

She sat there for a good 30 minutes, which in kid time equals a day-and-a-half. (And 7 years, 89 hours if you're a kid dog.) When Paris finished, she proudly called me over to see. Very nice, Paris. And when her grandmother came to visit later that evening, Paris immediately took her by the hand and led her to the taped-down ribbon sculpture.

Should I be concerned that not one, but two of my kids like to pass the time this way? Perhaps I am a carrier of the Compulsive Tape Disorder gene? Are my children destined to become gift wrappers at Nordstrom?

It took me half a decade, but I think I get it now. Justin and Paris were really holding up a mirror for me. "See, Mom? This is how what you do looks to us." Here I am thinking it is critical that I get my proposal to FedEx/redo the kids' closets/work on my Web site/finish this essay/ some pressing objective *du jour,* and oh, I take it very seriously, I pound away at it, you should watch me go. I devote time and energy and brain quadrants to it, and that's all well and good—after all, the entire Western civilization *is* counting on me to come through here—but to the next guy (and I believe his name is Gerald), my efforts seem as silly as adhering tape to a ukulele.

The kids aren't home. What's my idea of going wild? Cooking on the front burner with the pan handles facing out.

With Justin, and then later Paris, at that exact hour in their lives on that tiny X on their personal development grid charts, what they were doing was not only *not* pointless, it was very much the point.

***

Who knows why we, all of us, fill our time the way we do, what assignments and goals we concoct to carry ourselves from one moment to the next, what we expect it will all add up to. But poll your office or playgroup, and I bet most people will tell you that whatever it is they are doing, it's relatively important. Whether we're talking about work or leisure, I have no business judging someone else's time-passing choices. To the best of my recollection, Ghandi never called me and said, "Now, Amy—do you really think that the world will be better off because you made a run to K-Mart (undies, Band-Aids, coloring books, slotted spoon) and returned 20 e-mails this morning? Would you like to know how your previous 3 hours compare to mine?" No, he did his fasting, saving the world thing, and left me alone to do mine.

So after writing and thinking about the above, you'd think I'd have been supportive when, a few days later, the following dialogue occurred.

MILES: Are we almost home?
ME: Yes, we'll be home in a few minutes.
MILES: How high should I count?
ME (*not thinking he'd really do it*): I don't know. Count to 200, Miles, and we'll be home.
MILES: 1, 2, 3, 4, 5, 6, 7, 8, 9, 10, 11, 12, 13, 14, 15, 16, 17, 18, 19, 20, 21, 22, 23, 24, 25, 26, 27, 28, 29, 30, 31, 32, 33, 34, 35, 36, 37, 38, 39, 40, 41, 42, 43, 44, 45, 46, 47, 48, 49, 50, 51, 52, 53, 54, 55, 56, 57, 58, 59, 60, 61, 62, 63,

64, 65, 66, 67, 68, 69, 70, 71, 72, 73, 74, 75, 76, 77, 78, 79, 80, 81, 82, 83, 84, 85, 86, 87, 88, 89, 90, 91, 92, 93, 94, 95, 96, 97, 98, 99, 100, 101, 102, 103, 104, 105, 106, 107, 108, 109, 110, 111, 112, 113, 114, 115, 116, 117, 118, 119, 120, 121, 122, 123, 124, 125, 126, 127, 128, 129, 130, 131, 132, 133, 134, 135, 136, 137, 138, 139, 140, 141, 142, 143, 144, 145, 146, 147, 148, 149, 150, 151, 152, 153, 154, 155, 156, 157, 158, 159, 160, 161, 162, 163, 164, 165, 166, 167, 168, 169, 170, 171, 172, 173, 174, 175, 176, 177, 178, 179, 180, 181, 182, 183, 184, 185, 186, 187, 188, 189, 190, 191, 192, 193, 194, 195, 196 (somehow we were actually pulling into the garage at this point), 197, 198, 199, 200.*

---

*I did actually type all these numbers. I was trying to get myself into that mindset, of being satisfied doing nothing but counting to 200. When I got to 124, I realized I could copy and paste 25 to 99, and then just add a 1 in front of them, and for a moment, I decided that that was cheating, that I was rushing the Zen experience, but then that moment passed.

Clearly, this counting is the verbal equivalent of the Scotch tape madness, am I right? For those few minutes, couldn't he have thought about school or looked at a book or calculated his fat gram intake for the day? But this counting, this mindless, grating counting. I tell you, if I were given the gift of 3 free minutes in the backseat, I could:

1. Write some thank you notes.
2. Think about what I'm going to say at my father-in-law's 65th birthday brunch. (*"Please come with a funny memory or anecdote."*)
3. Unscrunch all the dollar bills in my wallet, and put them back nice and flat, in order of value.
4. Clean the backseat.

Clearly, I've learned nothing. ■

Lollipop Tree

Our friends Carol and Brian woke up early one morning and tied hundreds of lollipops to the tree in their backyard. They then called a bunch of us with kids to come over and join their family in a celebration in honor of their fantastic "lollipop tree," which, as anyone could see, had magically just come into full bloom.

For a few sacred minutes, watching those children jumping for joy, picking lollipops off the tree, shrieking with delight and wonder, all was well with the world.

lesson eleven

Touch the Sock

KNOCKING ON WOOD AND OTHER PRAYERS

I have two modes: sleeping and running late. In fact, come to think of it, that's what I want on my tombstone: *She's running late.*

So it's sometime in the year 2000, it's mid-morning, and I'm running late.

I do have an alibi. (If nothing else, children are always good for an alibi. *I'm so sorry we can't make it to the Bar Mitzvah 'n' Rodeo, my son woke up with . . . a clubfoot.*) The truth is that Miles was throwing up all night. Apparently, I missed the *Good Housekeeping* issue with the tip about not giving your child pancakes for breakfast, three Oreos for a snack at school, pizza and cake at a birthday party after school, and then an entire cantaloupe for dinner.

So when poor Miles finally got it out of his system, it was dawn, and we both fell asleep for a few hours. This put me in the position of having to start getting ready immediately upon waking, which, of course, is exactly what I did not do. Instead, I (tempo allegro) played with the kids, shuffled around some papers on the kitchen counter, eyed the clock, did something very crucial I'm sure, tested the laws of space and time just a bit more, and then finally went upstairs to shower. At that point, I had to leave the house, let's see . . . 6 minutes ago.

When I'm finally dressed and moderately presentable, I race downstairs and start throwing stuff into my backpack. I'm stressing out because I have too much crap and it's not all going to fit, dramatic sigh. I need a shopping bag to put some of my materials in—how pathetic and unprofessional, walking into this event with wet hair and a crinkly shopping bag. And my jeans are a little tight. That's really the problem here, isn't

I don't have all the answers. And when I do have one, I forget which question it belongs with.

it? My jeans are tight. Everything would be okay if only I didn't feel my stomach pressing against the waistband. I would be like, yes, okay, I am running late and am not the most together person in the world, but my jeans are fitting nicely, a bit loose even, everything's cool.

And at that moment, Paris wants me to go get her shoes. Here is a transcript of our exchange:

PARIS: Mommy, can you go get my shoes?

MOM: I can't get your shoes, Paris. I'm late. Can *you* go get your shoes?

PARIS: Please, Mommy. It's really important to me.

MOM: Paris, I can see your shoes right outside. They're right on the porch where you left them. Go get them, and I'll be right here waiting.

PARIS: Okay. (*Paris goes and gets her shoes. They are outside, right on the porch where she left them. At this time, Mom is throwing things into her backpack. Her jeans look a little tight.*) I got my shoes, Mommy.

MOM: Good job, Paris. Now Mommy has to go. I'll see you later, okay? I love you, I'll see you later.

PARIS: Wait, Mommy. Come here and touch my sock.

MOM: What? Touch your sock? Why do you want me—I can't touch your sock, Paris. I have to go. I'm so late. Oy, look what time it is. I'm really late.

PARIS: Please, Mommy. Touch my sock. (*Mom is thinking, "Why on Earth does she want me to touch her sock? Something is really wrong with my daughter."*) It's so warm. Come here, feel. (*Mom remembers "That's right, she left her shoes and socks out on the porch and the sun is so strong this morning, her socks must be warm from the sun."*)

And suddenly it all came down to this one moment. It was a quick zoom in on the sock, everything else in the room and in most of North America was now out of focus, irrelevant. Paris's lips were moving in slow motion, but no sound was coming out.

Touchhhhhhhhhhhhhhhhhhhhhhhhhhhhhhh the-e-e-e-e-e-e-e-e-e-e-e-e-e-e-e-e-e-e-e-e-e-e-e-e sockkkkkkkkkkkkkkkkkkkkkkkkkkkkkkkkkkkkkkkkkk

In short, my daughter's current and future sense of well-being was riding on this one decision.

If I don't touch the sock . . .

- I'll be out the door a few seconds earlier.
- I'll be holding my ground, some sort of statement about how I can't always accommodate her every whim.
- I'm not *that* good of a mom.
- She'll be upset for a minute, and then get over it just as quickly; or she'll be upset and actually *never* get over it.

If I touch the sock . . .

- No matter how busy I am, I know how to stop and smell the roses/touch the sock.
- I'm a really good mom.
- Sharing this warm sock moment with Paris ensures that she will grow up to be a

kind, happy, well-adjusted, bilingual neurosurgeon.

This ridiculous brain banter from a woman with 17 years of schooling and who made it to the state science fair in eighth grade (an experiment involving Fibonacci numbers and a chambered nautilus . . . fascinating). I know the above does not constitute logical thinking. Then why? What's going on here? Why *really* do I feel compelled to touch this piece of warm cloth?

Because to do so gives me hope. It gives me hope.

I don't know what I'm doing half the time. Don't know if all my decisions and efforts and love will tally up in a way that means my children will walk away from the carnival with the jumbo stuffed animal. I do what I can, what is in my power, but there are just so many other factors at work: things that are predetermined at birth; things that happen at school; things that happen in the in-between spaces; things I can't even fathom yet; things I'm unintentionally doing all wrong. That which is beyond my control, beyond my understanding, beyond the horizon, shrivels me.

***

In my younger years, crumpling up a piece of paper, I'd bargain, "If this goes into the wastebasket, I'll pass the test," or "He'll call me back," or just generally, "Everything will be okay." Making the basket may or may not have been the reason that a blind date turned into a second phone call, which turned into a marriage. But who knows what would have happened if I hadn't taken the shot?

When these pivotal occasions present themselves, when I find myself in a face-off with the bigness of life, I figure, what chance does a 5'1" mortal have, really, if she doesn't have a few sock-touchings under her belt?

MOM: You're right, Paris, your sock is so nice and warm. ■

Grocery List

Punchlist for Contractor

Questions for Parent/Teacher Conference

PHONE MESSAGES

Ladies, please claim the following undelivered phone messages, taken by various husbands. . . .

Janice called. Loves the sweater.

Megan called: a boy
Connor, 7 lb. 8 oz.
Her number at hosp.
312-932-1800
rm 136

DINA CALLED

Mrs (?) called from school.
Did you forget about conference?

Vince from Nordstrom called about your lost wallet;
will hold it for you at the customer service desk.

The kids will be waiting for you at the south entrance to
the mall, not the north like they said.

Some producer called. Would you
fly to Chicago in the a.m. to talk to
Oprah's book club?

Your mother called.

Lauren says happy birthday from your one friend who has never missed calling you on your birthday in 34 years.

Howard called. Do NOT go to the airport. The client is flying here instead.

Sasha Called -

URGENT!!! Found a donor with same blood type! Call within 6 hours.

Your mother called.

Patti called. How's the 21st of next month for dinner?

Margaret called -
~~Fou~~ Found the antique poster you've been looking for for 18 years. Tracked one down from a dealer in Switzerland. It's the last one in the edition! Page her at once.

Corrections

On page 63, the author didn't know what she was talking about.

On page 108, the author said her son Justin was 3 years old at the time. He was actually 3¼.

In 1996, when Miles brought home a painting from school, the author said, "Wow, Miles! That is fantastic, so great, I love it!" What she should have said, in a much more matter-of-fact way, according to various articles, was, "Look at that—a yellow sun and a purple tree. It makes me feel like going to the park."

During a phone conversation in 1997, the author told her mother that everything was great, fine. What she meant to say was, "I hate you for having four children and making it all look so easy. And my left nipple is infected."

Last night, after the author put the boys to bed, she let Paris stay up until 10:30 P.M. She should have put her to bed at 9:00; 9:20 at the latest.

Tomorrow the author is going to say something to her children that she's said many times before. Maybe it will be something in the car about remembering their manners at their friend's house, or something about how she hopes he/she has a good time and how she loves him/her very much, and this will annoy the child to no end. What she will mean to say is, "Bye."

In the future, the author will disappoint her children, make a bad decision, go against her gut, give in when she shouldn't have, not give in when she should have, go out of the house looking like *this,* look at her child the wrong way, talk on the phone when she should have hung up and spent time with her child, not watch a child jump on one leg when she said would. What she means to do is the right thing. ■